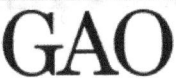

United States Government Accountability Office

Report to Congressional Requesters

I0426181

May 2012

VA DIALYSIS PILOT

Increased Attention to Planning, Implementation, and Performance Measurement Needed to Help Achieve Goals

To access this report electronically, scan this QR Code.

Don't have a QR code reader? Several are available for free online.

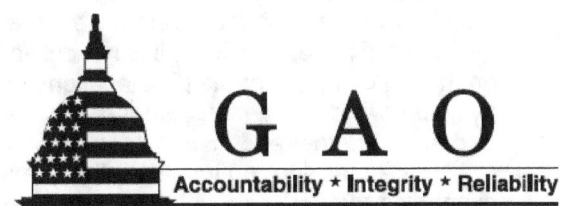

GAO-12-584

GAO
Accountability * Integrity * Reliability

Highlights

Highlights of GAO-12-584, a report to congressional requesters

VA DIALYSIS PILOT

Increased Attention to Planning, Implementation, and Performance Measurement Needed to Help Achieve Goals

Why GAO Did This Study

Veterans diagnosed with end-stage renal disease—a condition of permanent kidney failure—represent one of the most resource-intensive patient populations at VA. These veterans are often prescribed dialysis, which is a life-saving and relatively expensive medical procedure that removes excess fluids and toxins from the bloodstream. VA began developing its Dialysis Pilot in 2009 with four goals: (1) improved quality of care, (2) increased veteran access, (3) additional medical research opportunities, and (4) cost savings. Through this pilot, VA will establish four VA-operated outpatient dialysis clinics in communities surrounding select VA medical centers by the end of fiscal year 2012 using start-up funding provided by VA Central Office. Pilot locations are expected to achieve cost savings and to repay their start-up funding. GAO examined VA's planning and early implementation efforts for the Dialysis Pilot, and how VA plans to evaluate the pilot.

GAO reviewed relevant VA documents, including those related to pilot location selection and cost estimation, and spoke with VA officials responsible for overseeing the Dialysis Pilot and representatives from all pilot locations.

What GAO Recommends

Among other actions, GAO recommends that VA improve its Dialysis Pilot by providing guidance for start-up fund repayment, as well as developing an evaluation plan that includes performance measures for the pilot locations. VA concurred with GAO's recommendations and provided an action plan to address them.

View GAO-12-584. For more information, contact Randall B. Williamson at (202) 512-7114 or williamsonr@gao.gov.

What GAO Found

GAO found a number of weaknesses in the Department of Veterans Affairs' (VA) execution of the planning and early implementation phases of the Dialysis Pilot. These weaknesses involved pilot location selection, cost estimation practices, and cost savings calculations that could collectively limit the achievement of the pilot's goals. Specifically, VA did not do the following:

- **Appropriately document its pilot location selection process**. VA did not maintain a clear and transparent pilot location selection process; it did not document how its criteria for pilot location selection were applied to all 153 VA medical centers (VAMC) or why substitutions in pilot locations were made. However, VA officials reported that several criteria, including dialysis patient prevalence and average treatment costs, were used to select the pilot locations in Durham and Fayetteville, North Carolina; Philadelphia, Pennsylvania; and Cleveland, Ohio.

- **Produce consistent and comparable cost estimates for pilot locations**. VA did not complete consistent and comparable cost estimates for the four pilot locations. Specifically, GAO found several cases where pilot locations did not complete reliable cost estimates because they made changes to formulas and assumptions of the Dialysis Pilot cost estimation model, which was developed by VA systems redesign engineers.

- **Provide clear and timely guidance on start-up fund repayment and cost savings calculations**. VA did not provide Veterans Integrated Service Network and VAMC officials with clear and timely written guidance or instructions on how to pay back start-up funds, or how to calculate cost savings generated by the pilot locations.

VA Central Office has not yet determined how it will achieve its goals for the Dialysis Pilot or created clear performance measures for the pilot locations. Previously, GAO found that leading public sector organizations take three steps to improve their performance and help their organizations become more effective: (1) define a clear mission and goals, (2) measure performance to gauge progress toward achieving goals, and (3) use performance information as a basis for decision making. While VA has defined a clear mission and goals for the Dialysis Pilot, it has only made limited progress in the remaining two steps. In March 2012, VA reported that it was in the early stages of establishing an agreement with a leading university research center to conduct an evaluation of the Dialysis Pilot; however, no target dates were provided for when this evaluation would begin or what aspects of the Dialysis Pilot it would evaluate. Because VA has not yet developed an evaluation plan or defined performance measures for pilot locations, it is not collecting consistent and reliable information on the performance of the pilot locations and thus may not have this information available when it is time to either make midcourse corrections to the Dialysis Pilot or decide whether and how to open additional VA-operated outpatient dialysis clinics. VA officials also told GAO they have developed a limited plan for expanding the Dialysis Pilot despite not having access to performance information on the existing four pilot locations.

_____ United States Government Accountability Office

Contents

Abbreviations

CMS	Centers for Medicare & Medicaid Services
ESRD	end-stage renal disease
VA	Department of Veterans Affairs
VAMC	Veterans Affairs medical center
VHA	Veterans Health Administration
VISN	Veterans Integrated Service Network

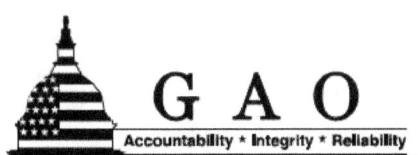

United States Government Accountability Office
Washington, DC 20548

May 23, 2012

Congressional Requesters

Veterans diagnosed with end-stage renal disease (ESRD)—a condition of permanent kidney failure—are one of the most resource-intensive patient populations the Department of Veterans Affairs' (VA) health care system serves. To treat the effects of ESRD, veterans with the disease are often prescribed dialysis, which is a life-saving medical procedure that removes excess fluids and toxins from the bloodstream.[1] Veterans diagnosed with ESRD must receive dialysis treatments for the rest of their lives unless they receive a kidney transplant. These treatments are time intensive for veterans and relatively expensive for VA. Dialysis typically requires veterans to undergo three outpatient treatments per week that each last about 4 hours. Due to VA's limited dialysis capacity in its own facilities, VA most commonly provides these dialysis treatments to veterans by referring them to non-VA outpatient dialysis clinics in their local communities through VA's fee basis program.[2,3] In fiscal year 2011, VA referred about 9,600 veterans to fee basis providers for dialysis treatments at a cost of about $314 million, up from about 6,900 veterans at a cost of about $133 million in fiscal year 2008.

To help address these rising costs, VA began developing its Dialysis Pilot in 2009. Through this pilot, VA will establish four VA-operated outpatient dialysis clinics in communities surrounding select VA medical centers (VAMC) by the end of fiscal year 2012. VA officials expect these new clinics will reduce the number of veterans referred to fee basis providers for dialysis treatments. Ultimately, VA believes the Dialysis Pilot will lead

---

[1]In this report, we use the term dialysis to describe hemodialysis—the most common form of dialysis treatment provided in the United States. VA provides dialysis as part of the medical benefits package it provides to all veterans enrolled in its health care system—a full range of hospital and outpatient services, prescription drugs, and noninstitutional long-term care services. See 38 C.F.R. § 17.38.

[2]Outpatient dialysis clinics are freestanding clinics that are typically located in convenient areas, such as shopping centers, and vary in the number of patients served. These clinics make these chronic treatments accessible to those who need them.

[3]Through its fee basis program, VA can pay for veterans to receive care from non-VA providers in the community for certain health care services that it is not capable of providing in its own medical facilities—such as dialysis treatment.

GAO-12-584 VA Dialysis Pilot

to the development of a business model with a mission of providing more veterans' dialysis treatments in VA facilities rather than through the fee basis program. To meet this mission, VA set four goals for the Dialysis Pilot: (1) to improve the quality of dialysis care veterans receive, (2) to increase veterans' access to dialysis care, (3) to provide additional dialysis research opportunities, and (4) to achieve cost savings for VA-funded dialysis treatments.

Congressional requesters expressed interest in the analysis VA performed to determine the cost-effectiveness of providing more veterans' dialysis treatments in VA-operated facilities. This report examines (1) VA's early planning and implementation efforts for the Dialysis Pilot and (2) how VA plans to evaluate the Dialysis Pilot.

To examine VA's early planning and implementation efforts for the Dialysis Pilot, we reviewed relevant VA Central Office, Veterans Integrated Service Network (VISN), and VAMC documents related to (1) pilot location selection, (2) cost estimation, and (3) pilot location start-up funding.[4] We also interviewed VA Central Office, VISN, and VAMC officials involved with the Dialysis Pilot—including officials from each VISN and VAMC operating a pilot location, the Veterans Health Administration's (VHA) Chief Business Office, the VHA Dialysis Steering Committee, the Dialysis Workgroup, and VA systems redesign engineers.[5] In addition, we analyzed VA's key decision-making tools—including the cost estimation models used to assess pilot costs—for each Dialysis Pilot location and the pilot as a whole. We also analyzed VA's data on dialysis fee basis expenditures. We verified these data with VA officials and found information derived from analysis of these expenditure data to be sufficiently reliable for our purposes.

---

[4]Each VISN is responsible for the day-to-day management of facilities within its network.

[5]The VHA Chief Business Office oversees the development of administrative processes, policy, regulations, and directives associated with the delivery of VA health benefit programs. The VHA Dialysis Steering Committee includes VA clinicians and officials who assess and assist in the management of the delivery of dialysis services for veterans enrolled at VA. The Dialysis Workgroup was created to research, design, and implement VA's Dialysis Pilot. VA's systems redesign engineers work at one of VA's Veterans Engineering Resource Centers. These centers support collaboration between researchers, systems redesign engineers, and clinicians to improve VA health care delivery.

To examine VA's plans to evaluate the Dialysis Pilot, we reviewed relevant VA and VISN documentation of key pilot plans and meetings—including business plans, implementation plans, approval documents, and meeting minutes. We also spoke with officials from VA Central Office and all three VISNs and four VAMCs operating pilot locations regarding (1) reporting responsibilities and expectations for the Dialysis Pilot and (2) any ongoing or planned evaluations of the Dialysis Pilot.

We conducted this performance audit from September 2011 to May 2012 in accordance with generally accepted government auditing standards. Those standards require that we plan and perform the audit to obtain sufficient, appropriate evidence to provide a reasonable basis for our findings and conclusions based on our audit objectives. We believe that the evidence obtained provides a reasonable basis for our findings and conclusions based on our audit objectives.

Background

VHA oversees VA's health care system, which includes 153 VAMCs organized into 21 VISNs. Each VISN is charged with the day-to-day management of the VAMCs within its network. VA Central Office decentralized its budgetary, planning, and decision-making functions to the VISN offices in an effort to improve accountability and oversight of daily facility operations. However, VA Central Office maintains responsibility for monitoring and overseeing both VISN and VAMC operations.

Providing Dialysis Treatments to Veterans

Veterans may elect to have their dialysis treatments through VA or Medicare but cannot receive dialysis benefits from both simultaneously. In 2008, there were over 18,000 veterans enrolled in VA's health care system diagnosed with ESRD who required dialysis treatments.[6] Of these enrolled veterans, about two-thirds elected to receive their dialysis treatments through VA. However, VA treated less than half of these veterans in VAMC-based dialysis clinics because of capacity limitations and other factors, such as long distances veterans may have to travel to

---

[6]See Corrigo Health Care Solutions, LLC, *Purchase of Non-VA Hemodialysis Treatments*, a report prepared at the request of the Department of Veterans Affairs, Veterans Health Administration, January 30, 2009. The VHA Chief Business Office awarded a contract to Corrigo Health Care Solutions, a professional services firm, to complete this study on VA's ability to purchase dialysis services both now and in the future.

the VAMC.[7] This limited internal capacity and other factors resulted in most of these veterans receiving their dialysis treatments through VA's fee basis program. Through VA's fee basis program, veterans can select any dialysis provider, as long as their chosen provider accepts VA's established payment rate for dialysis treatment. Currently, fee basis rates differ by VISN; however, several VISNs are currently paying for dialysis treatments through several multi-VISN-negotiated agreements with dialysis providers. Under these agreements, per-treatment costs for these VISNs currently range from $248 to $310. Veterans who elect to have their dialysis treatments provided through VA—either in VAMCs or through the fee basis program—may not incur any out-of-pocket expenses.

The remaining one-third of all veterans enrolled in VA's health care system who were diagnosed with ESRD, in fiscal year 2008, elected to have their dialysis treatments paid for by Medicare.[8] The veteran can select any Medicare-certified dialysis provider that accepts Medicare payment and there are few, if any, restrictions on this choice since all major dialysis providers accept individuals covered by Medicare. Medicare reimburses dialysis providers 80 percent of a specified per-treatment base bundled rate—about $230 in 2011—and beneficiaries or private insurance companies are responsible for the remaining 20 percent.[9] For veterans who elect to have their dialysis treatments paid for by Medicare, the remaining 20 percent may be an out-of-pocket expense that was about $7,600 per year in 2008, because VA is not authorized to pay these out-of-pocket expenses incurred by veterans covered by Medicare.

---

[7]See Corrigo Health Care Solutions, LLC, *Non-VA Hemodialysis Treatments*. At the end of fiscal year 2008, VA operated 64 VAMC-based dialysis clinics that treated both veterans in need of acute inpatient dialysis treatments and veterans receiving outpatient chronic dialysis treatments for ESRD.

[8]See Corrigo Health Care Solutions, LLC, *Non-VA Hemodialysis Treatments*. Medicare covers dialysis treatment for most individuals with ESRD regardless of age. Medicare coverage generally begins in the fourth month after they start dialysis. If an individual entitled to Medicare because of ESRD is covered by a commercial health insurance plan, the commercial plan is the primary payer and Medicare is secondary for the first 30 months of Medicare entitlement, after which Medicare becomes the primary payer. See 42 U.S.C. § 1395y(b)(1)(C).

[9]Medicare pays dialysis providers a single rate for providing dialysis treatment and certain related items and services, which is a common form of Medicare payment known as bundling.

| Development of the Dialysis Pilot | In 2009, VA began developing the Dialysis Pilot to build its in-house capacity to provide dialysis treatments to veterans in response to several issues, including the following: |

- **Rising numbers of veterans needing dialysis.** A VA-funded study found that the number of veterans requiring dialysis treatments was projected to increase 6 percent from fiscal year 2008 to fiscal year 2015 and the number of veterans receiving these dialysis treatments from community providers through the fee basis program was projected to increase 16 percent.[10]

- **Rising costs of providing dialysis through the fee basis program.** The same VA-funded study also found that VA's fee basis per-treatment costs were projected to increase about 59 percent from $337 per treatment in fiscal year 2008 to $535 per treatment in fiscal year 2015.[11]

- **Unsuccessful efforts to achieve lower reimbursement rates with fee basis dialysis providers.** Another VA-funded study found that if VA adopted Medicare rates, set by the Centers for Medicare & Medicaid Services (CMS), for outpatient dialysis treatments, it would reduce its dialysis fee basis expenditures by 39 percent resulting in projected cost reductions from fiscal year 2011 through fiscal year 2020 of about $2 billion.[12] As a result of this study, VA Central Office instructed VISN directors to begin using Medicare rates as the prevailing reimbursement rate for fee basis dialysis treatments in 2009. However, the major fee basis dialysis providers did not agree to provide dialysis treatments to veterans through VA's fee basis program at these reduced rates.[13] This resulted in VA continuing to

---

[10]See Corrigo Health Care Solutions, LLC, *Non-VA Hemodialysis Treatments.*

[11]See Corrigo Health Care Solutions, LLC, *Non-VA Hemodialysis Treatments.*

[12]See Kennell and Associates, Inc., *Report on Medicare Pricing of Outpatient Services*, a report prepared at the request of the Department of Veterans Affairs, Veterans Health Administration, November 18, 2009.

[13]The dialysis industry is very concentrated, with many facilities owned and operated by a few organizations. For example, about 61 percent of the approximately 5,600 dialysis facilities nationwide are owned by three large organizations.

pay for these treatments according to previously established rates, which are typically higher than Medicare rates.[14]

In response to these issues, VA Central Office charged VISN 6, a VISN with a significant volume of veterans who require dialysis treatments, with establishing a dialysis workgroup to evaluate VA's options for dialysis treatment delivery.[15] The Dialysis Workgroup—led by officials from VISN 6, with representatives from VA Central Office and the VHA Chief Business Office and others with financial and clinical expertise—met in 2009 to discuss various options for providing dialysis care for veterans. This workgroup identified several options VA could take to build its internal capacity to provide dialysis treatments to veterans and identified several ways VA could address the rising costs of dialysis care provided through the fee basis program, including (1) building dialysis units in leased space in communities surrounding select VAMCs, (2) purchasing modular dialysis units, (3) modifying existing space in selected VAMCs to expand or build dialysis units, and (4) negotiating pricing agreements with select dialysis providers to allow VAMCs to pay a lower rate for fee basis dialysis treatments.[16]

In March 2010, after discussing these options and exploring potential solutions, the Dialysis Workgroup began designing the Dialysis Pilot as an effort to build VA's capacity to provide dialysis treatments to veterans in VA-operated facilities and reduce fee basis costs. The Dialysis Workgroup projected that the Dialysis Pilot would result in a 5-year cost savings of about $33 million by operating four outpatient dialysis clinics that could each treat 48 veterans a week. The Dialysis Pilot was approved by the Under Secretary for Health in August 2010 and by the Secretary of Veterans Affairs in September 2010. The final four pilot locations selected by the Dialysis Workgroup were Durham and Fayetteville, North Carolina; Philadelphia, Pennsylvania; and Cleveland,

---

[14]In December 2010, VA amended its regulations to apply CMS rates to all non-VA inpatient and outpatient medical services, including dialysis. See 75 Fed. Reg. 78,901 (Dec. 17, 2010) (amending 38 C.F.R. §§ 17.52, 17.56).

[15]VISN 6 oversees eight VAMCs in North Carolina, Virginia, and West Virginia and serves a veteran population with a high prevalence of ESRD.

[16]Modular dialysis units are buildings or trailers that are predesigned and can be installed on VAMC property. These units are designed to meet the standards of several health care accrediting and surveying entities, including CMS, state agencies, and The Joint Commission.

Ohio. Each of these locations was provided approximately $2.5 million in start-up funding by VA Central Office to establish an outpatient dialysis clinic with 12 dialysis stations that could treat 48 veterans per week. VA Central Office expected this start-up funding would be repaid by the pilot locations. (See app. I for more information on the current status of each pilot location.)

The pilot locations in Durham and Fayetteville, North Carolina, began treating veterans in June 2011. The Philadelphia, Pennsylvania, pilot location is scheduled to open in May 2012, and the Cleveland, Ohio, pilot location is scheduled to open in September 2012.

Planning and Early Implementation Phases of the Dialysis Pilot Had Significant Weaknesses

There were a number of weaknesses in VA's execution of the planning and early implementation phases of the Dialysis Pilot that collectively could limit the achievement of its goals. Specifically, weaknesses in pilot location selection, cost estimation practices, and cost savings calculations could hamper the Dialysis Pilot's effectiveness.

VA's Pilot Location Selection Process Was Not Transparent or Appropriately Documented

While the Dialysis Workgroup reported using several criteria to select the Dialysis Pilot locations and documented some of these criteria in the approval documents for the Dialysis Pilot, it did not document how these criteria were applied or whether it assessed all 153 VAMCs for potential inclusion in the Dialysis Pilot. According to GAO internal control standards, clearly documenting key information is necessary to ensure that appropriate internal controls for communicating and recording decision-making activities are in place.[17] According to Dialysis Workgroup officials, the Dialysis Workgroup began its pilot location selection process by identifying 13 potential pilot locations using several criteria, including (1) the number of veterans receiving outpatient dialysis treatments living within a 30-mile radius or a 30-minute drive of a VAMC, (2) a VAMC's potential to achieve cost savings by operating a pilot location, and (3) the

[17]See GAO· *Standards for Internal Control in the Federal Government*, GAO/AIMD-00-21.3.1 (Washington, D.C.: November 1999). Standards for internal control in the federal government state that information should be recorded and communicated to management and others within the agency that need it in a format and time frame that enables them to carry out their responsibilities.

perceived level of dialysis-related clinical expertise available at each VAMC.[18] Dialysis Workgroup officials told us that the final four pilot locations in Durham, Fayetteville, Philadelphia, and Cleveland were all ultimately selected because they had a high number of veterans receiving dialysis treatments and, in some cases, had access to high-quality clinical expertise. However, no documentation was provided by VA discussing how these criteria were applied to all 153 medical centers and why Durham, one of the final four pilot locations, was omitted from the list of 13 potential pilot locations when it clearly met these selection criteria.[19] In addition, VA officials from the Dialysis Workgroup whom we spoke with could not recall complete details regarding the pilot location selection process that occurred in 2009, including whether additional VAMCs were assessed against the various criteria. As a result, it is not possible for VA or an external party to definitively determine if there were any other VAMCs that could have been viable pilot locations beyond the 13 considered by the Dialysis Workgroup.

The transparency of the pilot site selection process was further compromised by the manner in which the Durham VAMC was selected as a pilot location. Dialysis Workgroup officials did not document their rationale for selecting this VAMC—a site not included in the original 13 potential pilot locations—as one of the four final pilot locations. According to Dialysis Workgroup officials, the VAMC in Salisbury was originally selected as one of the four final pilot locations; however, this VAMC was undergoing managerial changes at that time and the VAMC in Durham, located in the same VISN, was selected as a replacement pilot location. In April 2012, Dialysis Workgroup officials reported that the Durham VAMC's high number of veterans receiving dialysis and nephrology expertise also contributed to its selection as one of the four final pilot locations. However, VA did not document either the initial

---

[18]The 13 potential pilot locations were VAMCs located in Ann Arbor, Michigan; Augusta, Georgia; Cleveland, Ohio; Dublin, Georgia; Erie, Pennsylvania; Fayetteville, North Carolina; Los Angeles, California; Kansas City, Missouri; Loma Linda, California; Philadelphia, Pennsylvania; Phoenix, Arizona; Sacramento, California; and Salisbury, North Carolina.

[19]In April 2012, Dialysis Workgroup officials told us that how the pilot location selection criteria were applied was documented in a series of e-mails between VA systems redesign engineers. However, these e-mail messages did not contain a transparent and clear description of the application of these criteria and included some information that contradicts other documentation of the selection process provided by the Dialysis Workgroup.

selection of the VAMC in Salisbury as a pilot location or the rationale for why the VAMC in Durham was a better final selection for the Dialysis Pilot than one of the other 13 potential pilot locations that was not selected. The lack of documentation on this particular selection further reduced the transparency of the decision-making process.

VA Central Office officials do not have complete information about how or why pilot locations were selected because key decisions and the rationale behind them were not documented. Such documentation of decision-making processes is necessary to ensure that VA decision makers have access to relevant, reliable, and timely information and could follow a rigorous and fair decision-making process for this critical aspect of the Dialysis Pilot. The lack of documentation related to a key planning decision—such as the complete process used to select pilot locations—limits VA's ability to access this information in the future, evaluate the success of the Dialysis Pilot, and make decisions about how best to expand the pilot to additional locations.

VA Did Not Produce Consistent and Comparable Cost Estimates for Pilot Locations

It is not possible to determine whether pilot locations completed reliable cost estimations because these estimates are not consistent and comparable. This will limit VA's ability to determine if the Dialysis Pilot has met its mission to reduce the cost of dialysis treatments paid for by VA. Reliable cost estimates are necessary to ensure that pilot location costs are comparable across the four pilot locations.[20] Generating reliable and comparable cost estimates prior to opening the pilot locations was critical to the early implementation of the Dialysis Pilot in order to ensure that appropriate site-specific baseline cost estimates were generated that would allow VA to evaluate the cost of the Dialysis Pilot and ensure that any cost savings generated by the pilot locations could be accurately calculated. The importance of thorough and reliable cost estimation processes was included in VA's own business analysis of the Dialysis Pilot, which stated that pilot locations were intended to use the same cost estimation methodology to facilitate uniformity and ensure that all pilot locations produced reliable information.

---

[20]See GAO/AIMD-00-21.3.1. Standards for internal control in the federal government state that information should be recorded and communicated to management and others within the agency that need it in a format and time frame that enables them to carry out their responsibilities.

To its credit, the Dialysis Workgroup worked with VA systems redesign engineers to develop a sophisticated cost estimation model to help VISN and VAMC officials estimate costs for their pilot locations. VA systems redesign engineers built the cost estimation model using validated research as the foundation for its general baseline cost estimates. The cost estimation model included information on several aspects of establishing and operating an outpatient dialysis clinic—including equipment costs, leased-space costs, staff costs, and veteran travel costs.[21] (See fig. 1.)

Figure 1: Selected Components of the Dialysis Pilot Cost Estimation Model

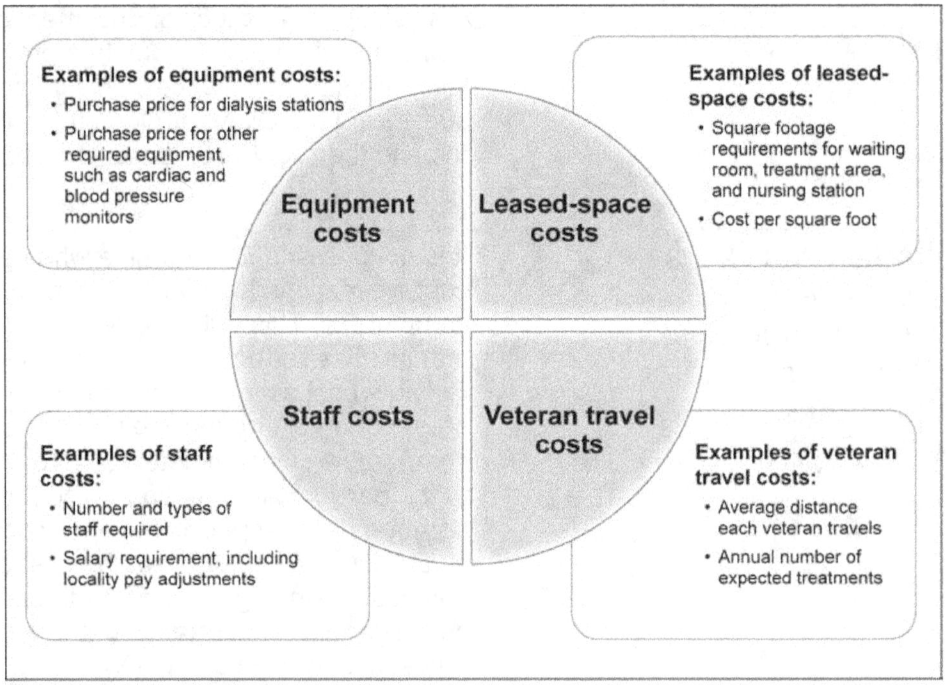

Examples of equipment costs:
- Purchase price for dialysis stations
- Purchase price for other required equipment, such as cardiac and blood pressure monitors

Examples of leased-space costs:
- Square footage requirements for waiting room, treatment area, and nursing station
- Cost per square foot

Equipment costs

Leased-space costs

Staff costs

Veteran travel costs

Examples of staff costs:
- Number and types of staff required
- Salary requirement, including locality pay adjustments

Examples of veteran travel costs:
- Average distance each veteran travels
- Annual number of expected treatments

Source: GAO.

---

[21]VA reimburses some veterans for travel expenses associated with their care and treatment. Eligibility for these travel reimbursements is determined by several factors, including a veteran's service-connected disability rating, pension status, and annual income.

Despite this effort to build a robust model for estimating Dialysis Pilot costs, VA did not maintain proper control over the cost estimation model following its release for use by VISNs and VAMCs. While there were designated areas in the cost estimation model for each pilot location to enter its specific cost inputs, a VA systems redesign engineer we spoke with explained that the formulas in the cost estimation model should not be customized by pilot locations. These formulas were validated by VA systems redesign engineers and were meant to remain constant across all pilot locations to ensure that comparable and consistent cost estimates were produced. However, VA Central Office requested that the cost estimation model be fully customizable—including all cost inputs and formulas—in order to encourage pilot locations to use the model. Because the model was fully customizable, some pilot locations both appropriately altered their pilot location-specific inputs and inappropriately altered the formulas that were intended to remain constant. As a result of the inappropriately altered formulas, final cost estimates for the four pilot locations are inconsistent and do not include comparable information.

We found several inconsistencies in pilot locations' use of the cost estimation model, including the following:

- **Not all pilot locations used validated formulas for developing cost estimates**. We found that not all pilot locations used the validated formulas developed by VA systems redesign engineers to calculate their cost estimates. For example, Philadelphia's cost estimation model did not use the validated formula for calculating the pilot location's equipment costs. While the validated equipment cost formula included a patient transport cardiac monitor for each dialysis pilot location, the Philadelphia pilot location's model omitted this equipment from its calculation. Also, instead of using the validated formulas, the Cleveland pilot location deleted some formulas related to annual patient demand and leased-space costs and replaced them with specific numeric values. As a result of these changes, some of Cleveland's cost estimations cannot be confidently compared with those from the other three pilot locations because it is unclear what the location used to calculate these numeric values. Consistent use of the cost estimation model and its validated formulas is necessary to ensure that the cost estimations of each pilot location can be compared and evaluated.

- **Pilot location capacity changes**. Two pilot locations increased the capacity of their outpatient dialysis clinics, despite the fact that the Dialysis Workgroup specifically established clear capacity limits and the cost estimation model was developed for these specific capacity limits. According to the Dialysis Workgroup and the Dialysis Pilot approval document signed by the Secretary of Veterans Affairs, each pilot location's capacity was limited to 12 dialysis stations that could provide up to 48 veterans with dialysis treatments each week.[22] However, the Fayetteville pilot location increased its capacity from 12 to 16 dialysis stations and the Cleveland pilot location increased its capacity from 12 to 20 dialysis stations. These capacity increases were not validated by VA systems redesign engineers, and as a result, it is unclear how these changes may affect the efficiency of these pilot locations. In addition, it is unclear whether these capacity increases were approved by VA Central Office since the size of these two pilot locations is larger than what was originally approved by the Secretary of Veterans Affairs.

According to Dialysis Workgroup officials, pilot location-specific baseline cost estimates were included in VA's own business analysis of the Dialysis Pilot. However, the baseline cost estimates included in this document are unreliable for the following reasons:

- The baseline cost estimates included in VA's business analysis of the Dialysis Pilot are based on the assumption that all pilot locations will be limited to 12 dialysis stations. However, the Cleveland and Fayetteville pilot locations currently have considerably more dialysis stations, with 20 and 16 dialysis stations, respectively.

- The baseline cost estimates included in VA's business analysis of the Dialysis Pilot were generated prior to the cost estimation model's distribution to pilot locations for customization. Therefore, these estimates do not account for the pilot location-specific customization of several model inputs, such as actual leased-space costs. During

---

[22]The Dialysis Workgroup's review of private sector dialysis models and dialysis operations of academically affiliated medical centers found that 12 dialysis stations is the minimum required size for a dialysis unit to achieve operating efficiencies. According to VA's business analysis of the Dialysis Pilot, this finding is consistent with the private sector staffing standard of one dialysis technician for every 4 patients and one registered nurse for every 12 patients. As a result of these findings, the Dialysis Workgroup recommended that the four pilot locations be limited to 12 dialysis stations.

the site-specific customization process, several of the costs associated with these customizable inputs increased significantly due to either changes in pilot location size or other factors. For example, the Cleveland pilot location's customized model includes about $400,000 in annual lease expenses, while the baseline cost estimate for Cleveland's lease expenses from VA's business analysis is only about $220,000.

VA Did Not Provide Clear and Timely Guidance to Pilot Locations on Start-up Fund Repayment and Cost Savings Calculations

VA Central Office officials did not provide VISN and VAMC officials with clear and timely written guidance or instructions on how to pay back start-up funds or how to calculate cost savings from the Dialysis Pilot. VA Central Office provided a total of approximately $10 million in start-up funding for the Dialysis Pilot to the three VISNs associated with the pilot locations. Each pilot location received about $2.5 million in start-up funding to establish its outpatient dialysis clinic. Pilot locations are expected to achieve cost savings through the outpatient dialysis clinics and to repay their start-up funding. Specifically, the memorandum approving the Dialysis Pilot signed by the Secretary of Veterans Affairs and the Under Secretary for Health states that pilot location start-up funds are to be repaid in two equal payments in fiscal year 2012 and fiscal year 2014.

A lack of communication—including ongoing discussions, reporting, and guidance—regarding the repayment of pilot location start-up funds could make it difficult for VA and external parties to determine if the pilot locations are making reasonable progress toward repaying these funds and realizing cost savings from the Dialysis Pilot.[23] VISN and VAMC officials reported a lack of clarity about how Dialysis Pilot start-up funds must be repaid. Specifically, officials from two of the three VISNs associated with pilot locations—VISNs 4 and 10—told us that they have not discussed the repayment of their pilot locations' start-up funding with VA Central Office. Similarly, officials from the VAMCs associated with the two operational pilot locations acknowledged their understanding that start-up fund repayment would likely be included as part of their cost

---

[23]See GAO/AIMD-00-21.3.1. Standards for internal control in the federal government state that information should be recorded and communicated to management and others within the agency that need it in a format and time frame that enables them to carry out their responsibilities.

savings calculations, but told us that they were not aware of any specific agreements or plans for repayment.[24]

In addition, while the Dialysis Workgroup provided pilot locations with 5-year cost savings projections and articulated plans for calculating actual cost savings in a document that was published prior to the approval of the Dialysis Pilot, VISN officials we spoke with were uncertain about how cost savings would be calculated. According to VA's own business analysis of the Dialysis Pilot, actual cost savings will be calculated by comparing the cost per treatment at each pilot location to actual fee basis per-treatment rates for each pilot location's corresponding VAMC.[25] This document also states that cost saving calculations will be a collaborative effort between pilot location leadership, VA researchers, and the VHA Chief Business Office. However, VISN officials stated that while they expect that the cost savings from their pilot locations will be examined, they did not receive written guidance about how cost savings will be calculated. Given the lack of specific and timely guidance to VISN and VAMC officials on the calculation of cost savings, officials at the pilot locations may not use the same methodology to track these savings.

VA's Dialysis Pilot Has a Stated Mission but Lacks Clearly Defined Performance Criteria and an Evaluation Plan

VA Central Office has not yet determined how it will define success for the Dialysis Pilot or created clear performance measures linked to the four Dialysis Pilot goals. When other leading public sector organizations are engaged in efforts to improve their performance and help their organizations become more effective—similar to VA's goals for the Dialysis Pilot—we found that these organizations commonly take three steps: (1) define a clear mission and goals, (2) measure performance to gauge progress toward achieving goals, and (3) use performance information as a basis for decision making.[26]

---

[24]Only the pilot locations in Durham and Fayetteville, North Carolina are currently operational. The pilot locations in Philadelphia, Pennsylvania; and Cleveland, Ohio; are scheduled to open in May and September 2012, respectively.

[25]Each pilot location's cost per treatment will be calculated using VA's standard cost assignment methodology contained in its Decision Support System.

[26]GAO, *Executive Guide: Effectively Implementing the Government Performance and Results Act*, GAO/GGD-96-118 (Washington, D.C.: June 1996).

Step 1—Defining a clear mission and goals. VA has completed the first of these steps by defining a clear mission and goals for the Dialysis Pilot. Specifically, the Dialysis Workgroup noted that the Dialysis Pilot would allow VA to develop a cost-effective business model that could be used to optimize VA's resources and increase its capacity to provide dialysis treatment to veterans. This workgroup also outlined four goals of the Dialysis Pilot: (1) improved quality of care, (2) increased access for veterans, (3) additional dialysis research opportunities, and (4) cost savings for VA-funded dialysis treatments. Through the participation of its membership in developing this mission and these goals, the Dialysis Workgroup was able to incorporate the input of several VA internal stakeholders—including VA Central Office representatives, VISN leadership, clinical experts with experience treating veterans with ESRD, and VA systems redesign engineers. This process included a thorough assessment of VA's options for providing dialysis treatments to veterans—including the resources, equipment, and staffing needed to operate a cost-effective outpatient dialysis clinic.

Step 2—Measuring performance to gauge progress. Despite its success in defining a clear mission and goals for the Dialysis Pilot, VA has not developed a clear plan for evaluating the pilot. Specifically, while two pilot locations (Durham and Fayetteville) began treating veterans in June 2011, VA has not yet begun an evaluation of the establishment and management of the pilot locations—including causes for opening delays, operating challenges, or the sufficiency of start-up funding. Previously, we found that developing sound evaluation plans before a pilot program is implemented can increase confidence in results and facilitate decision making about broader applications of the pilot.[27] In March 2012, the VHA Chief Business Office reported that VA is in the early stages of establishing an agreement with a leading university research center to conduct an evaluation of the Dialysis Pilot; however, no target dates were provided for when this evaluation would begin or what aspects of the Dialysis Pilot beyond cost-effectiveness it would evaluate.

---

[27]See GAO, *Limitations in DOD's Evaluation Plan for EEO Complaint Pilot Program Hinder Determination of Pilot Results*, GAO-08-387R (Washington, D.C.: Feb. 22, 2008), and *Tax Administration: IRS Needs to Strengthen Its Approach for Evaluating the SRFMI Data-Sharing Pilot Program*, GAO-09-45 (Washington, D.C.: Nov. 7, 2008).

In addition, VA Central Office has not developed a cohesive strategy for evaluating the Dialysis Pilot and has not yet formally defined its criteria for measuring the performance of the pilot locations or the success of the Dialysis Pilot in general. Several potential performance measures could be used to measure the pilot locations' progress toward the achievement of each Dialysis Pilot goal:

- **Improved quality of care**. Officials from the Dialysis Workgroup told us that quality assurance outcomes, specifically those used by CMS to certify outpatient dialysis clinics, could be used to assess pilot locations.[28] These metrics would likely help VA assess the quality of dialysis care provided by the pilot locations.

- **Increased access for veterans**. Dialysis Workgroup officials told us that patient satisfaction information could be used to assess pilot locations. This potential metric could help determine if the pilot locations increased veterans' access to dialysis care.

- **Additional dialysis research opportunities**. In its business analysis of the Dialysis Pilot, the Dialysis Workgroup recommended that VA fund a 4-year research study to evaluate the quality of care at all pilot locations and identify best practices in veteran dialysis care. According to this business analysis, the findings of this study would enable VA to develop an evidence-based strategy for veteran dialysis care that ensures veterans receive the highest quality of care.

- **Cost savings for VA-funded dialysis treatments**. In its business analysis of the Dialysis Pilot, the Dialysis Workgroup suggested that pilot locations could use the cost estimation model to calculate cost savings generated by the pilot locations by comparing the cost of providing dialysis at each pilot location to the cost of providing this treatment through fee basis providers. However, this potential performance metric may be limited by VA's failure to maintain control

---

[28]State survey agencies monitor the quality of dialysis care by periodically evaluating dialysis organizations' adherence to Medicare's Conditions for Coverage for ESRD Facilities. These conditions for coverage are the minimum health and safety rules that dialysis facilities participating in Medicare must meet. 42 C.F.R. Part 494. In particular, the conditions for coverage direct dialysis facilities to develop, implement, and maintain an ongoing internal quality oversight program that focuses on indicators related to improved health outcomes. 42 C.F.R. § 494.110.

over the cost estimation model or provide sufficient guidance to pilot locations about how to properly use it.

Because VA has not yet developed an evaluation plan or formally defined performance measures for pilot locations, it does not have access to consistent and reliable information on the performance of the pilot locations and may not have this information accessible when it is time to either make midcourse corrections for the Dialysis Pilot or decide whether and how to open additional VA-operated outpatient dialysis clinics.

Step 3—Using performance as a basis for decision making. Despite not having fully developed performance measures for assessing the pilot locations, VA has already begun planning for the expansion of the Dialysis Pilot, which should not occur until after VA has defined clear performance measures for the existing pilot locations and evaluated their success. Specifically, a member of the VHA Dialysis Steering Committee told us that the committee has already developed a limited plan for expansion of the Dialysis Pilot. However, this plan does not incorporate the results of a performance assessment for the existing four pilot locations. In addition, VA systems redesign engineers have begun developing three additional cost estimation models despite not having fully evaluated the effectiveness of the cost estimation model used in the Dialysis Pilot.[29] Taken together, these two actions indicate that VA is beginning to make decisions about the future of the Dialysis Pilot and the cost estimation model, even though VA decision makers currently lack critical performance information on the existing four pilot locations.

Conclusions

To its credit, VA developed the Dialysis Pilot as a potential way of addressing the rising cost and utilization of fee basis dialysis treatments among veterans. Through the Dialysis Pilot, VA intends to test the viability of increasing its capacity to provide dialysis treatments in VA-operated outpatient dialysis clinics. VA set four goals for its Dialysis Pilot: (1) improve quality of care, (2) increase access for veterans, (3) provide additional dialysis research opportunities, and (4) achieve cost savings for VA-funded dialysis treatments. While these are commendable goals, there were weaknesses in VA's planning and early implementation of the Dialysis Pilot that if not corrected, will make it difficult to determine

---

[29]These new models analyze the feasibility of VAMCs expanding existing on-site dialysis, gastroenterology, and polysomnography (sleep study) units.

whether the Dialysis Pilot has met its goals and will provide cost-effective care if expanded. Specifically, VA did not conduct a transparent and well-documented pilot location selection process, provide clear and timely guidance to participating VISNs and VAMCs on key financial aspects of the Dialysis Pilot, or articulate clear performance measures for pilot locations. We believe that VA can rectify these weaknesses, but must act prior to full implementation of the four pilot locations to ensure that the Dialysis Pilot is not compromised and can serve as an effective demonstration effort. Moreover, until VA has reliable data, we believe it would be unwise for VA to expand the Dialysis Pilot beyond the current four pilot locations, as doing so may risk investing resources inappropriately.

Moving forward, we believe four critical areas should be addressed. First, VA must clearly document the selection process it used to identify the existing four pilot locations and may use to identify any future pilot locations. VA relied on a decentralized and ad hoc selection process to choose the existing four pilot locations and failed to properly document the results of this key decision-making effort. Such inattention to documenting critical decisions results in a lack of transparency and weakens the credibility of the Dialysis Pilot.

Second, VA needs to ensure that changes to its cost estimation model are reviewed by knowledgeable staff. This step is necessary to ensure that this model produces comparable data for all pilot locations that can serve as an accurate basis for evaluating the financial success of the Dialysis Pilot. To date, pilot locations altered existing formulas and model assumptions, which resulted in cost estimation data with questionable reliability that may limit VA's ability to compare results consistently across the pilot locations.

Third, VISN and VAMC officials need specific guidance for the repayment of Dialysis Pilot start-up funds and the calculation of cost savings realized from the pilot locations. To date, VA Central Office has not articulated its expectations regarding these two critical aspects of the Dialysis Pilot. Without a clear understanding of the terms for start-up fund repayment, it is difficult for VA or external entities to determine if the four pilot locations are making significant progress toward repaying these funds and generating cost savings that can be used to offset the cost of treating the projected increased number of veterans who will need dialysis treatment in the coming years.

Finally, VA must develop clear and measurable performance criteria that can be consistently applied to evaluate the Dialysis Pilot. Despite defining the mission and goals for the Dialysis Pilot, VA has not developed a plan for evaluating its success or developed performance measures to track pilot locations' progress toward meeting its stated mission and goals. An effective evaluation plan and clear performance measures are needed to help ensure that the Dialysis Pilot operates in an environment of accountability.

Recommendations for Executive Action

In order to increase VA's attention to planning, implementation and performance measurement of the Dialysis Pilot we are making five recommendations.

To improve VA's communication related to the Dialysis Pilot, we recommend that the Secretary of Veterans Affairs direct the Under Secretary for Health to ensure that key decisions made regarding pilot location selection and efforts to continue or expand the Dialysis Pilot are clearly documented.

To ensure that reasonable cost estimates are created for the Dialysis Pilot and other similar programs, we recommend that the Secretary of Veterans Affairs direct the Under Secretary for Health to restrict or evaluate changes made to cost estimation models at the VISN and VAMC levels that affect pilot development and analysis.

To ensure that start-up funds are repaid and cost savings are accurately calculated for the Dialysis Pilot, we recommend that the Secretary of Veterans Affairs direct the Under Secretary for Health to develop written guidance about expectations for the repayment of start-up funds and how the cost savings generated by the four pilot locations should be calculated.

To ensure that VA Central Office effectively evaluates the Dialysis Pilot, we recommend that the Secretary of Veterans Affairs direct the Under Secretary for Health to take the following two actions:

- Develop an evaluation plan that outlines how the Dialysis Pilot will be assessed and provides target dates for the completion of this assessment.

- Develop clear measures for assessing the performance of the four Dialysis Pilot locations in key areas—including quality, access, and cost.

Agency Comments and Our Evaluation

VA provided written comments on a draft of this report, which we have reprinted in appendix II. In its comments, VA generally agreed with our conclusions, concurred with our recommendations, and described the department's plans to implement each of our five recommendations. VA did not provide any technical comments.

In its general comments, VA noted that it has established a comprehensive strategic plan for chronic kidney disease and dialysis services; however, a copy of this strategic plan was not provided as part of VA's response to the draft report. According to VA, this plan incorporates aspects of several of our recommendations. In addition, VA stated that it is in the process of developing longer-range plans for the expansion of dialysis services, including establishing additional freestanding outpatient dialysis clinics similar to the current four pilot locations. We support VA's efforts to carefully analyze its delivery of dialysis services to veterans, including the most cost-effective method of providing these life-saving medical treatments, and make reasoned decisions based on a thorough evaluation of its current pilot locations. In this regard, we continue to believe that it is unwise to establish additional freestanding outpatient dialysis clinics until the current four pilot locations are fully evaluated and VA rectifies the weaknesses we identified in this report.

In its plan for addressing our recommendations, VA stated that it is developing a plan for the Dialysis Pilot that will address three of our recommendations related to (1) the documentation of Dialysis Pilot key decisions, including the selection of future pilot locations; (2) the creation of reasonable cost estimates for pilot locations; and (3) guidance for the repayment of start-up funding and cost savings calculations. According to VA, this plan will ensure better communication and documentation of decisions for future pilot site selections; more rigorous oversight of cost estimation tools and analysis of financial and clinical outcomes; and a thorough analysis of start-up fund repayment, including whether VA will reverse its decision to require repayment of these funds. VA's anticipated completion date for these actions is July 1, 2012.

Finally, to address our remaining two recommendations, VA intends to develop a detailed evaluation plan for the Dialysis Pilot by July 1, 2012. According to VA, this plan will include specific criteria, target dates, and activities that must occur throughout the remainder of the pilot. VA intends to use this plan to periodically review and evaluate the Dialysis Pilot. In addition, VA described its efforts to significantly enhance the decision-making tools used for the Dialysis Pilot, including the cost estimation model. VA reported that these enhancements will include more rigorous accounting for facility costs, such as those for staffing and equipment. In addition, VA plans to task its systems redesign engineers with assessing pilot locations' performance using metrics for cost, access, and quality.

We are sending copies of this report to the Secretary of Veterans Affairs, appropriate congressional committees, and other interested parties. In addition, the report is available at no charge on the GAO website at http://www.gao.gov.

If you or your staff have any questions about this report, please contact me at (202) 512-7114 or williamsonr@gao.gov. Contact points for our Offices of Congressional Relations and Public Affairs may be found on the last page of this report. GAO staff who made major contributions to this report are listed in appendix III.

Randall B. Williamson
Director, Health Care

List of Requesters

The Honorable Patty Murray
Chairman
The Honorable Richard Burr
Ranking Member
Committee on Veterans' Affairs
United States Senate

The Honorable Jeff Miller
Chairman
Committee on Veterans' Affairs
House of Representatives

The Honorable Bill Johnson
Chairman
Subcommittee on Oversight and Investigations
Committee on Veterans' Affairs
House of Representatives

The Honorable Michael Michaud
Ranking Member
Subcommittee on Health
Committee on Veterans' Affairs
House of Representatives

Appendix I: Status of VA Dialysis Pilot Locations

Table 1 provides additional information on the current operating status of the four Dialysis Pilot locations at the Department of Veterans Affairs (VA) medical centers (VAMC) in Durham, North Carolina; Fayetteville, North Carolina; Philadelphia, Pennsylvania; and Cleveland, Ohio.

Table 1: Status of Dialysis Pilot Locations as of March 2012

Pilot VAMC location	Anticipated capacity	Current operating status	Implementation challenges pilot locations reported
Fayetteville	Sixteen dialysis stations serving 64 veterans	Operational since June 2011	• **Planning and building issues**. The pilot location's leased space required that floor drains be installed, which delayed the progress of constructing the outpatient dialysis clinic.
Durham	Twelve dialysis stations serving 48 veterans	Operational since June 2011	• **Difficulty finding an appropriate clinic location**. Identifying an appropriate location and entering into a contract and lease for the outpatient dialysis clinic took longer than anticipated. • **Equipment testing**. The pilot location's water purification system, a necessary component of the dialysis process, needed additional testing prior to the opening of the outpatient dialysis clinic.
Philadelphia	Twelve dialysis stations serving 48 veterans	Not yet operational; scheduled to become operational in May 2012	• **Contracting challenges**. The pilot location's first contract for leased space was canceled due to zoning issues that the contractor did not disclose. A second location and a new contractor were identified and construction of the pilot location is under way.
Cleveland	Twenty dialysis stations serving 80 veterans	Not yet operational; scheduled to become operational in September 2012	• **Difficulty finding an appropriate clinic location**. The VAMC initially planned to incorporate the pilot location into an existing VAMC enhanced-use lease project.[a] However, VA Central Office determined that the clinic could not be added to this enhanced-use lease. A lease for space in a new location is pending.

Source: GAO.

[a]Under VA's enhanced-use lease program, VA property may be leased for non-VA uses, provided those uses are compatible with or benefit the department's mission. VA requires lessees either pay rent or offer VA "in-kind" consideration.

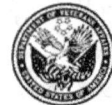

DEPARTMENT OF VETERANS AFFAIRS
Washington DC 20420

May 14, 2012

Mr. Randall Williamson
Director, Health Care
U.S. Government Accountability Office
441 G Street, NW
Washington, DC 20548

Dear Mr. Williamson:

The Department of Veterans Affairs (VA) has reviewed the Government Accountability Office's (GAO) draft report, *"VA DIALYSIS PILOT: Increased Attention to Planning, Implementation, and Performance Measurement Needed to Help Achieve Goals"* (GAO-12-584) and generally agrees with GAO's conclusions and concurs with GAO's five recommendations to the Department.

The enclosure specifically addresses GAO's five recommendations and provides an action plan for each. VA appreciates the opportunity to comment on your draft report.

Sincerely,

John R. Gingrich
Chief of Staff

Enclosure

Enclosure

Department of Veterans Affairs (VA) Comments to
Government Accountability Office (GAO) Draft Report:
*VA DIALYSIS PILOT: Increased Attention to Planning, Implementation, and
Performance Measurement Needed to Help Achieve Goals*
(GAO-12-584)

GAO Recommendation 1: To improve communication related to the Dialysis Pilot, we recommend that the Secretary of Veterans Affairs direct the Under Secretary for Health to take the following action: ensure key decisions made regarding pilot location selection and efforts to continue or expand the Pilot are clearly documented.

VA Response: Concur. The Veterans Health Administration (VHA) is developing a Dialysis pilot plan to ensure that the reasons for any future pilot site selections are more clearly documented and communicated. The plan will include greater transparency over the existing sites and any expansion of the pilot. The anticipated completion date of the plan is July 1, 2012.

GAO Recommendation 2: To ensure reasonable cost estimates are created for the Dialysis Pilot and other similar programs, we recommend that the Secretary of Veterans Affairs direct the Under Secretary for Health to take the following action: restrict or evaluate changes made at the VISN and VAMC levels to cost estimation models that impact pilot development and analysis.

VA Response: Concur. VHA's Dialysis Plan will include more rigorous oversight and management of the pilot, including strict controls on all aspects of cost estimation tools and analysis as well as financial and clinical outcomes. VHA has planned and will soon initiate an agreement for an external review of the pilot, comparing the VHA program with external dialysis programs for quality, cost, and other outcomes. This review will be included in VHA's overall strategic decision model for providing end-stage renal disease (ESRD) services in the future. The anticipated initiation date of the agreement is July 1, 2012.

GAO Recommendation 3: To ensure start-up funds are repaid and cost savings are accurately caluculated for the Dialysis Pilot, we recommend that the Secretary of Veterans Affairs direct the Under Secretary for Health take the following action: develop written guidance about expectations for the repayment of start-up funds and how the cost savings generated by the four pilot locations should be calculated.

VA Response: Concur. VHA's plan will provide for a more rigorous and structured deployment of the pilot that will include detailed cost documentation and analysis. The plan includes an analysis of potential repayment of start-up funds and consideration if repayment of start-up funds will be required. See the response to Recommendation 4 for more detail. The anticipated completion date of the plan is July 1, 2012.

2

Enclosure

Department of Veterans Affairs (VA) Comments to
Government Accountability Office (GAO) Draft Report:
*VA DIALYSIS PILOT: Increased Attention to Planning, Implementation, and
Performance Measurement Needed to Help Achieve Goals*
(GAO-12-584)

To ensure that VA Central Office effectively evaluated the Dialysis Pilot we recommend
that the Secretary of Veterans Affairs direct the Under Secretary for Health to take the
following two actions.

Recommendation 4: Develop an evaluation plan that outlines how the Dialysis Pilot
will be assessed and provides target dates for the completion of this assessment.

VA Response: Concur. VHA will utilize multiple assessment factors. Several of these
factors very clearly use quantitative criteria, such as evaluating planned vs. expected
efficiencies; patient quality; and patient satisfaction. VHA will evaluate the dialysis pilot
results in relation to expectations where they are available.

However, the pilot process also ensures VHA gains visibility over certain areas that may
not be as subject to quantitative assessment and may not be clearly anticipated in the
plans for a pilot. For instance, in this pilot VHA has learned about the level of effort
required to implement a stand-alone clinic, to include specifications to be included in
plans, dedication of management staff, etc. These lessons, though not subject to
quantitative analysis, are important in order to adequately plan any expansion. VHA
expects to evaluate both the quantitative results as well as qualitative information.

A detailed evaluation plan, including specific criteria, target dates and activities that
must occur during the future of the dialysis pilot, is being developed. Periodic reviews
at specific milestones will be a component of this evaluation to ensure VHA has ongoing
analysis of the pilot.

Additionally, during the time that the GAO was engaged in its analysis, VHA had begun
significant enhancements to its estimating models. These enhancements include
applying more rigor to facility cost factors, treatment staffing frameworks, staff shifts,
equipment investments, and related costs. In addition to the enhanced cost estimation
toolset, VHA established criteria to evaluate sites using factors such as density of
Veterans requiring dialysis services, proximity to a VA health care center, and other
factors. VHA is identifying the level of investment required, ongoing operating costs and
identified return on investment (as compared with estimated contract costs). VHA is
using these increasingly detailed estimation techniques to assess the economic
feasibility of efficiently extending VHA dialysis services to more Veterans. Because
these changes were not finalized at the time of the review, they were not shared in
detail with the GAO review team. VHA officials have begun discussing these with GAO
team members and will continue to do so. The anticipated completion date of the plan
is July 1, 2012.

3

Enclosure

Department of Veterans Affairs (VA) Comments to
Government Accountability Office (GAO) Draft Report:
*VA DIALYSIS PILOT: Increased Attention to Planning, Implementation, and
Performance Measurement Needed to Help Achieve Goals*
(GAO-12-584)

Recommendation 5: Develop clear measures for assessing the performance of the
four Dialysis Pilot locations in key areas—including quality, access, and cost.

VA Response: Concur. VHA has developed success criteria and will use these criteria
to begin measuring results of each pilot location. With the more structured approach
now in place, the systems redesign staff will be responsible for analysis of cost, access
and quality data metrics and report those metrics through appropriate VHA committee
structure. The anticipated completion date for the development of the measures is July
1, 2012.

4

**Department of
Veterans Affairs**

Memorandum

Date: MAY 1 5 2012

From: Under Secretary for Health (10)

Subj: GAO Draft Report VA DIALYSIS PILOT Increased Attention to Planning, Implementation, and Performance Measurement Needed to Help Achieve Goals

To: Chief of Staff (00A)

1. I have reviewed the draft report and appreciate the Government Accountability Office (GAO) review of this important topic. The Veterans Health Administration (VHA) concurs with the GAO recommendations and appreciates GAO's identification of areas for improvement in regard to documentation of reasons for decisions, criteria for evaluation, and development of evaluation strategies.

2. Entering into the pilot for freestanding dialysis clinics, VHA developed initial dialysis service planning and pilot site evaluation methods to inform future dialysis strategy decisions. At that time, VHA recognized these methods would need to be expanded and enhanced, but VHA program managers sought to meet aggressive timelines for the freestanding dialysis pilots. VHA revised planning and analysis material, significantly enhancing estimation, analysis, and planning capabilities, prior to the delivery of the GAO's report. VHA established a comprehensive Chronic Kidney Disease and Dialysis Service Strategic Plan. This plan incorporates many of the recommendations made by the GAO. The freestanding dialysis pilots are being evaluated within the context of this much more robust planning and analysis context. VHA will ensure that each dialysis pilot will be evaluated against quantitative criteria in VHA's dialysis strategic plan. These pilots will generate valuable information about the expected efficiency gains from these pilots. Further, each pilot will assess clinical quality and patient satisfaction. VHA is also assembling additional valuable information about how to successfully stand up freestanding dialysis clinics, e.g. project planning, implementation staffing, leasing, procurement, and other issues. Notwithstanding the GAO's concerns about the selection of the clinic sites, the lessons learned from the pilot sites will enable VHA to assess the patient care and efficiency benefits of these clinics. I am confident that VHA will be able to draw solid conclusions from this pilot phase and will execute a transparent decision regarding any further expansion of dialysis services provided through freestanding clinics.

3. As indicated above, VHA began enhancement of its planning and estimating models while the GAO review was underway. VHA's dialysis plan *now* encompasses greater rigor in estimating facilities cost factors, staffing models for treatment centers, staff shifts, and equipment investments. VHA has a site evaluation methodology that employs factors such as density of Veterans requiring dialysis services, proximity to VA health care centers, as well as a

Page 2

GAO Draft Report GAO 12-584 "VA DIALYSIS PILOT: Increased Attention to Planning,
Implementation, and Performance Measurement Needed to Help Achieve Goals"

make-buy tool identifying requirements and associated costs such as staffing,
equipment, clinical supplies, construction or leasing, pharmacy, laboratory,
operations, and beneficiary travel. This site evaluation methodology is being
used to develop longer-range plans for deployment of additional dialysis clinic
sites that will meet Veterans' needs.

4. Combining the estimation tools and the site plans has enabled VHA to identify
the level of investment required, ongoing operating costs and return on
investment (as compared with estimated contract costs). VHA will be using the
improved estimation techniques to assess the economic feasibility of efficiently
extending VHA dialysis services to more Veterans. As these strategies are
developed, VHA officials will share the plans with GAO.

5. Thank you for the opportunity to review the draft report. Attached is the
complete corrective action plan for the report's recommendations. If you have
any questions, please contact Linda H. Lutes, Director, Management Review
Service (10A4A4) at (202) 461-7014.

Robert A. Petzel, M.D.

Attachment

Appendix III: GAO Contact and Staff Acknowledgments

GAO Contact	Randall B. Williamson, (202) 512-7114 or williamsonr@gao.gov
Staff Acknowledgments	In addition to the contact named above, Marcia A. Mann, Assistant Director; Kathleen Diamond; Katherine Nicole Laubacher; Rebecca Rust; and Malissa G. Winograd made key contributions to this report. Lisa Motley provided legal support.